NAILA GAFFAR

Self-Care Ritual for Women

A Guide on the best practices to heal your inner soul, body and mind

This book was professionally typeset on Reedsy.
Find out more at reedsy.com

Contents

1

Introduction:

Welcome to the Self-Care Ritual for Women! My name is Naila Gaffar and I'm very excited to be writing this book! I am looking forward to sharing some of the best self-care practices and tips that I have learned to help women like you and me create a daily self-care routine that energizes your soul while keeping you feeling your best.

The other reason I'm looking forward to writing this book is because now having a self-care ritual of my own, I can truly see the importance it has had on my health and well-being, especially my happiness and confidence. I want to help other women feel this way and show them that self-care is not a luxury but a necessity.

2

My Journey to Discovering Self-Care

A brief background about myself…I wasn't too familiar with the term self-care until a few years ago when I was in my freshman year of college. Just like every college student I was trying to balance school, assignments, work, social life, and additional responsibilities but was always overwhelmed and starting to experience burnout. I thought how would I be able to handle this for the next few years until I graduate I felt like I was just going through the motions but I wasn't really mentally there at that moment. One day when meeting up with a close friend they mentioned how ever since implementing self-care into their routine they were feeling like themselves again instead of feeling on the verge of a mental breakdown. I thought but how do you have the time? I barely have enough hours to sit and catch my breath. And wouldn't that require spending a lot of money on myself? Well, I was completely wrong. My friend explained that self-care doesn't equal blowing money but instead doing something or a couple of things for at least a few minutes out of the day that you enjoy like going for a walk or baking your favorite dessert. In other words, self-care is something that you need to make a priority since you can't pour from an empty cup.

3

Importance of Self-Care for Women

In today's world, women have many roles and responsibilities such as working, going to school, and caring for others along with additional stressors they may be facing throughout their busy lives. Sometimes taking time for themselves doesn't happen as these roles and responsibilities may cause them to put others' needs before their own. However, over time this can result in burnout, and things they used to look forward to doing don't bring them the same joy it once did. Additionally, they may feel that they are being selfish for taking time to do self-care or that it requires spending a large amount of money to do so but it is the exact opposite of that. Self-care doesn't need to be expensive or complicated, it can be something that you do for yourself on a daily basis that makes you feel good physically and mentally sometimes without spending any money.

This book may not include every single type of self-care practice out there as self-care is unique to each person but it can help to provide some ideas and tips for those who are looking to start or further their self-care journey. I'm simply here to provide you with the most condensed guide of the practices that fall under the eight types of self-care which are that are Emotional, Physical, Mental, Social, Spiritual, Practical, Professional, and Financial self-care without the need to search online or read 100s of pages to find what you are looking for.

This isn't the type of book that you have to read from start to finish. Instead, it's something that you can refer to when you need some inspiration or ideas. Let's say you are looking to do some Physical self-care but want to try something new then simply look at the table of contents and refer to "Physical Self-Care Practices". Or maybe you want some tips on how to schedule self-care throughout the day then simply refer back to the "Additional Tips for Self-Care" section. I like to have this book organized in a way that no matter what you are looking for in terms of self-care it can be found here.

With all of those things said, let's begin the journey into discovering the world of self-care!

4

Barriers and Limitations to Self-Care

Before talking about the different types of self-care I feel that it is important to briefly touch on barriers that prevent or limit someone from taking part in self-care activities. Some of these barriers include having feelings of selfishness or guilt for taking time for themselves, not having enough time due to a very busy schedule, lack of education about what self-care truly means, believing that self-care requires spending money (most self-care is free!), feeling like they are unworthy of self-care, and not having support from those around them such as at home or their workplace. While some may experience these situations, it's important to know that you deserve time for yourself even in the busiest of times and that self-care can be anything simple or small that you like to do and most of them don't require spending any money.

5

Emotional Self-Care

So let's begin with our first form of self-care which is known as emotional self-care. When you think of emotional self-care you may be thinking well isn't that something you do that makes you feel happy? Yes, it is but it's actually a little deeper than that. Doing something that makes you feel happy is important but we also need to focus on our ability to regulate all of the emotions that we experience regularly. Also, how we should cope with the difficult and challenging feelings we are presented with from certain circumstances. Additionally, emotional self-care involves taking the necessary steps to connect to our emotions and being able to process them in a way that is beneficial for our health and well-being. It is extremely important to spend quality time and attention working on this type of self-care as it can help you to develop stronger coping strategies to deal with unfortunate circumstances which can then increase your positive emotions such as happiness and feelings of joy. Some examples of practices that focus on emotional self-care include:

- Daily journaling

- Talking to a close friend, family member or therapist
- Reading positive affirmations
- Meditation
- Listening to your favorite music
- Setting personal boundaries
- Practicing mindfulness (gratitude)

Writing or journaling in a personal diary or notebook can be a great way to release all of the emotions you are feeling at the time by allowing you to organize your thoughts without having to speak out aloud to someone. When you are writing, be as creative as you like such as using drawings or scribbles to express your emotions as well. Listening to your favorite music or playlist at any point during your day can be a great way to release any tension or anxious emotions that you are experiencing and warn that it may result in your own personal dance party. Having someone that you can talk to who will always listen to what you have to say without judgment is an amazing way to express verbally how you feel whether it be a close friend, aunt/uncle, mom/dad, therapist, or counselor. Additionally, meditation helps to calm feelings of anxiety or worry that you have and the best part is that it can done anywhere that is peaceful to you such as outside in the sun, in a closed room, or at the beach. When we are feeling down, instead of focusing on what is going wrong, we should shift our focus to what good things we have in our lives. This is known as practicing gratitude which can help to lower our feelings of stress and anxiousness while appreciating the good things and people in our lives.

We also need to pay further attention to how we are speaking to ourselves daily, because if we are saying negative words and thoughts to ourselves then over time we continue to believe them. To prevent this unhealthy habit from forming, try practicing replacing any negative self-talk with positive and kind words.

6

Physical-Self Care

Mainly when someone hears the term self-care this is what they are mostly thinking of. Physical self-care is the act of doing something with your body to make you feel good physically. This can vary based on your lifestyle if you work a job where you are sitting down for the majority of the day you may want to do a more high-energy activity such as going for a walk with your dog or taking a workout class. Whereas someone who has a more physically demanding job may want to do something that doesn't require as much energy such as taking a calming bath, getting a massage, or their nails done. Some examples of practices that can promote physical self-care include:

- Going for a walk/run or to a workout class
- Taking a warm bubble bath
- Getting a facial or your nails done
- Taking a nap or going to sleep early
- Throwing your own personal dance party
- Nourishing your body with a diet of quality whole foods

- Keeping yourself hydrated with plenty of fluids
- Maintaining personal/oral hygiene

(This is not an exhaustive list, as there are many more ideas that you can do as well to practice physical self-care but be sure to do something that you enjoy!)

Now, some women may not have the time to get a facial or go to a workout class if their schedule doesn't allow but even doing something simple as doing your daily skincare, giving yourself a facial massage (using a gua-sha as a bonus), or brushing your teeth and hair can also be forms of physically caring for ourselves. A great way to maintain your oral hygiene is tongue-scarping with a tongue scraper and oil-pulling with coconut oil each morning. Incorporating healthy and balanced eating habits ensures that your body is getting all the nutrients it needs. Try incorporating more whole food sources such as protein, fruits, and vegetables into your diet. Moreover, including exercise in your daily routine can improve your physical well-being by releasing endorphins which in turn reduce cortisol (our stress hormones) and lead to a better physical appearance or increased energy. There are added benefits to doing physical self-care such as decreased stress, increasing your productivity and energy levels, prevention of diseases, and increased life expectancy.

7

Mental Self-Care

Self-care for our mental well-being involves taking additional actions to maintain a harmonious connection with our mind. This includes doing tasks that ensure our mind remains active and involved which are in the form of brain-enrichment activities. It's not about achieving a perfect mental state, but rather about recognizing and cultivating a compassionate bond with your own mind. Are you someone who struggles to wake up in the morning or to go to sleep at night? Do you ever feel overwhelmed or like your brain has become nonexistent after a busy day of work? Here are some mental self-care practices that you can implement in your daily life to enhance and re-energize your brain:

- Learning a new hobby (knitting, baking/cooking, gardening, dance lessons, poetry or creative writing)
- Taking some time off of social media
- Listening to podcasts (especially some about mental health/brain health)
- Reading a book

- Doing word puzzles
- Going to a museum or local art gallery
- Having a regular exercise routine
- Taking a walk
- Gardening

While these are some great activities to strengthen your brain, we shouldn't forget that mental self-care can also include working on regulating our thoughts and ideas. Also, establishing some personal boundaries between our close friends and family or with our work life. Even though we live in a time where Social Media is very prevalent in our lives and most of us spend many hours in the day scrolling and looking at other's lives, sometimes we need to take a step back from the screen and go do things in the moment with no selfie or post required. Getting exercise on a regular basis is the best way to allow your brain to release any tension while being able to increase your problem-solving skills. An example of this can be going for a morning or evening walk in your community or at a local park. Additionally, becoming involved in a new hobby can allow your mind to learn and adapt but eventually, it could become something that you do regularly when you have spare time. Some of my favorite hobbies I took up when starting my self-care journey were gardening and baking and they are two things that now I look forward to doing on a daily basis. Also, curling up with a hot cup of coffee or tea and a good book whether it be a classic or a new one can recharge your brain. Lastly, more and more podcasts have recently been coming out about older and newer subjects ranging from health and fitness to comedy and drama. They allow us to stay updated on current topics in the world while being very accessible so that you can listen in the comfort of your own home or your morning work commute.

8

Social Self-Care

Humans but specifically for the sake of this book women are always seeking out social interactions with others around them which also applies to those who are not always a big fan of interacting with others. Therefore, actively participating in social self-care, allows us to reinforce our bonds with others, which is essential to our well-being. Sometimes when our lives get busier than usual or additional responsibilities get added on to our already overwhelming schedule it causes us to reschedule or cancel our previously made plans with others. Of course, we could just do a video or phone call with one another which is more convenient but meeting in person and having that social interaction does wonders for both our bodies and brains. However, there are times that if it is in our best interest to say no to any plans then we should not feel guilt or shame for doing so as we are only human and sometimes we need a break to recharge. This has been particularly common in recent years, with many schools and workplaces adopting more online options. Even if you are someone who lives by themselves or feels that you do better without interacting with others socially just keep in mind that connecting with others is not a luxury but instead a necessity to our personal well-being! Some of my favorite social self-care practices include:

- Calling a family member or friend
- Hosting a Karaoke or game night with your friends
- Going on a date with your partner
- Curling up with your furry companion
- Going to the movies with friends
- Joining a friend for coffee
- Joining new clubs or groups to meet new people
- Using social media to stay in touch
- Attending a workout class
- Volunteering at a local daycare or senior center
- Sending a letter or card to a close friend or acquaintance

A simple and easy way to practice social self-care is by calling a friend or family member. This allows you to catch up on things happening in your lives, get some thoughts about some things that have been thinking about recently, or just talk about anything that comes to mind. It's a convenient way to connect with someone without leaving your home. Typically, social self-care is more focused on going out and getting involved in activities with others. Whether it's a weekly date night with your partner at a favorite restaurant or seeing a new movie at the theater with your friends, personal interaction is essential to us feeling more connected with those around us. This will lead our body to release endorphins which in turn can have mood-boosting effects on well-being such as our mood. It can even be something that you haven't done before like volunteering at an elderly care facility which allows you to meet new people while giving back to those in need. Maybe you are someone who loves doing activities that require moving your body and decides to attend a new workout class that you haven't been to before but end up enjoying it more than you thought. If you want to do something with others that doesn't require going somewhere, reach out to some of your friends nearby and see if they want to do a karaoke or trivia night at someone's home which can allow you to learn new things about one other. While all of these are great ways to practice social self-care, sometimes unfortunate circumstances happen like we get sick or become injured but that doesn't mean that we can't enjoy physical interaction. Using social media in a more conservative way by communicating with friends or family who don't live nearby or taking part in an online community forum are great ways to communicate with others when we are unable to leave our homes. One of my favorite practices that is quite simple to do on a regular basis is that if you do have a furry friend that wants some extra loving, grab a warm blanket and cuddle with them because even they need some self-care too.

Although social self-care means connecting and spending time with others, it can also mean the exact opposite. Are there some relationships with others that make you feel mentally exhausted or stressed? Do you feel like these connections to these individuals don't serve you the way they used to? Unfortunately, it may be time to go separate ways with that friend or family member as the purpose of your relationships is to fulfill and inspire you, not bring you down or make you feel mentally and physically worn out.

9

Spiritual Self-Care

This form of self-care may mislead you to think that you have to belong to a certain religious group or actively hold beliefs in one, but in reality, it can be beneficial to anyone whether religious, atheist, agnostic, or part of another belief system. Spiritual self-care can involve actions you take to establish and nourish a connection with your inner self. This is usually something that allows you to connect your inner spirit. For some, it can be carrying out practices that pay respect to a higher entity such as God, the Universe, or any guiding force that you hold beliefs in. Similarly, spiritual self-care is a fundamental tool for everyone even if you are struggling to feel more grounded in your daily routine. This can also be very helpful for those who have experienced a recent loss, have medical or financial challenges, or have any unexpected stresses that life throws our way. Some examples of these include:

- Connect with nature
- Meditation exercises
- Read inspirational quotes or positive affirmations

- Deep breathing exercises (doing 1-minute deep breaths throughout the day)
- Attend a worship service
- Prayer
- Spend 10 minutes doing a full-body scan technique to check in with your body
- Volunteer for a local cause in your community
- Eat a meal outside in the sun or sit on the grass
- Perform a random act of kindness
- Practice yoga or attend a yoga class
- Creating a vision/dream board for goals you want to achieve
- Going on a wellness retreat

It may seem like there are a lot of different ways to practice spiritual self-care but keep in mind that there is no wrong or right answer as to which activities to take part in since we are all unique and have different things that we enjoy. Connecting with nature and taking a walk in a local park are both ways to allow our minds to flow freely and to appreciate the small things around us. Even unexpected things like paying for the person's coffee ahead of you or holding the door open are little things that can make such a difference in someone's day and it most certainly doesn't go unnoticed. When we are feeling stressed or like things are spiraling out of control, a great way to calm ourselves is to incorporate daily deep breathing exercises. While there are numerous breathing exercises to choose from, I will not be going through all of them since this is meant to be a condensed guide but I will focus on how to do a basic deep-breathing exercise. Deep breathing is a great practice to do especially when you are having feelings of breathlessness as it ensures that air doesn't become stuck in your lungs and allows for you to breathe in fresh air. It can also promote feelings of calmness and control. First start by either standing or sitting (whatever position is comfortable), then move your elbows back a little to allow for your chest to rise, then take a deep breath in through your nose, hold your breath for at least a few seconds (start with 5 and work up to whatever you feel comfortable with), then gently exhale through your nose as you let out your breath. Doing this when we are feeling stressed or for 10 minutes each day (you can always work up to 20 minutes or more), can help to release any anxiety or tension that you are experiencing. During this exercise, it's highly encouraged to include imagery by closing your eyes and focusing on imagining something that makes you feel at peace. It is also recommended to have a focus word or a short phrase to repeat during this exercise that helps to reinforce that calm state.

You may be wondering how can I ensure that I can be successful in carrying out my spiritual self-care routine. Well, you can first start by trying to do these practices on a daily basis at whatever time during the day works for your schedule. Additionally, when doing activities such as prayer or meditation try to find a serene and quiet spot in your home for this purpose. One of my favorite ways to start the day on a positive note is to steer clear of checking my email or social media for the first hour of the day. During this one hour maybe spend it having your coffee outside while reading, making yourself a yummy breakfast, or doing a morning workout. Journaling in the morning and reading positive affirmations or mantras can additionally help set the tone for a productive day ahead. Another great option if your budget and schedule allow, is to attend a wellness retreat where you can be able to further connect with yourself on a spiritual level and interact with others that share similar beliefs.

10

Practical Self-Care

All steps that are taken to ensure that your fundamental needs are met while helping to reduce stress can be classified as practical self-care. It may sound silly but those little mundane things that you do on a regular basis like checking your mailbox, doing your laundry, or making your bed may be annoying at first but you end up feeling so much better after you do them. While these activities may not be as thrilling as others, they are more important than you think and shouldn't be overlooked. They help to keep your mental well-being in check while creating a feeling of relaxation and direction throughout our hectic lives. Practical self-care is especially beneficial to certain individuals such as young adults, college students, stay-at-home parents, caretakers, or anyone who finds it difficult to stay in a routine. Below, are some examples of practical self-care activities that most of us may do on a regular basis:

- Checking your mailbox
- Washing the dishes
- Straightening up your living area

- Preparing meals for the week
- Doing your laundry
- Scheduling doctor's appointments
- Making a to-do list for this week
- Laying out your clothes for the next day
- Going through your email inbox

Some of the most basic tasks are the ones that can make the biggest difference in our day. Like when we prepare our meals for the week, yes it takes a few hours out of our day and will result in a sink of dirty dishes to clean but now we have most of our food prepared so even on the busiest days of the week we can still enjoy a quality meal while spending hours in the kitchen. Really it's about making a sacrifice in the beginning whether that be big or small that pays off more in the end. Practical self-care can also be used to help form healthy and consistent habits that we can implement into our daily routine such as reducing our cell phone or screen time use, establishing better sleep habits like going to sleep early and waking up earlier or having time set aside daily to keep our living areas neat and less cluttered.

11

Professional Self-Care

If you are employed, then it is highly recommended for you to take time for professional self-care. When thinking about this form of self-care you may be wondering, How can I practice self-care while doing work? Or that I'm too busy at my job to do it but there are many ways to incorporate self-care in your workday. Implementing these activities can allow you to feel more in control and create a work-life balance in your profession. Maybe you are someone who doesn't enjoy their job or doesn't view it as being very demanding, but it is important for you to still include professional self-care in your day to avoid experiencing burnout in the future and to keep you motivated to reach your goals. If you recently are employed, have a job with overbearing hours, or are someone in charge who wants to provide additional resources for others in your workplace, please consider applying some of the practices listed below:

- Bringing your own lunch from home
- Going outside for breaks
- Eating lunch outside or with your co-workers

- Setting small, measurable daily goals for yourself
- Creating boundaries with your job responsibilities
- Avoid using your phone throughout the day (put it on airplane or do not disturb mode)
- Interacting with your co-workers
- Writing a to-do list for the day (include a lunch break!)
- Taking time off (mental health day, use PTO)
- Creating a workspace that fits your needs
- Avoid looking at your work email or computer after hours
- Enrolling in courses or working with a mentor to further your career goals

When you find activities or practices that help to better manage your physical and mental well-being in the workplace, this allows you to feel more grounded and calm throughout your day. By practicing self-care it helps to serve as a reminder to you that while you are an employee you are also human and that we need to take care of ourselves first. Whether it be scheduling your lunch break into your to-do list so that you can take time to enjoy your meal outside or creating small, measurable goals for yourself, these are great ways to increase your productivity. If you are someone who gets easily distracted at work or struggles with time management, try keeping your phone in an area that is out of sight either on airplane or do not disturb mode. Sometimes we don't want to admit it but a break is necessary to reset ourselves from a hectic work life. So the next time you need to take a mental health or personal day or use some of your paid time off don't feel guilty. Of course, whatever you decide to do with your time off such as scheduling appointments for your personal well-being or catching up on some errands that have been needing to get done can make all the difference. Most people feel much more energized after their time off and are able to come back to work refreshed and ready to take on the day. Even though we carry out many responsibilities at our job, we should not hesitate to decline any tasks that we are not meant to be doing. This may require you to put some boundaries into place and not be afraid to speak up or say no if you already have too much on your plate. Setting these personal boundaries is a great way to maintain a positive work-life balance that can impact your physical and mental health. This also allows you to get through your tasks for that day at a steady pace and be able to complete them by your deadline.

12

Financial Self-Care

This is another type of self-care that is not the most exciting but like practical self-care, it is necessary and important for us to do on a regular basis. Managing our personal expenses and ensuring that we are staying on track to meet our financial objectives is referred to as financial self-care. When practicing this form of self-care we can be more conscious of our spending habits to ensure that our bills are paid on time which can reduce financial-related stressors. Regularly checking in on bank accounts like any savings or investment accounts can allow us to be more aware in our decision-making which in turn can promote financial success over time. Some examples of ways to practice financial self-care include:

- Paying bills on time
- Meeting with a financial advisor
- Creating a budget that works for you
- Completing your yearly taxes
- Reviewing bank accounts on a daily basis
- Learning money management skills

- Creating measurable financial goals
- Paying off any outstanding balances

25

At first, many of these activities may feel daunting but over time as you implement them within your routine you may view them as very insightful to keeping you on top of your expenses and getting you closer to reaching desired financial objectives. When keeping a record of all expenses and income allows you to create a budget that works for your needs. Whenever you are unsure of something related to your finances, meeting with a financial advisor is a great way to receive guidance related to personal expenses and help you on your way to achieving your financial goals.

13

Additional Tips for Self-Care Planning

I f you have gotten to this point and are still wondering these are some great ideas but how can I implement them into my daily routine that is already packed, then you came to the right place. I wanted to provide some insightful tips on how to plan out your self-care even on the busiest of days, weeks, and months. What I first like to do is have a paper copy of a planner that I can write out all of the things that I know are happening for that week or month. Of course, plans change and appointments or meetings can be canceled but having somewhere where everything is written down, is extremely helpful. You don't have to use a paper or notebook planner, but use what works best for you such as a digital calendar that you can download onto your computer. After I write out everything, I will schedule my self-care as an appointment since you are most likely to hold yourself accountable for following through and least likely to cancel or reschedule it. Also if you have any other calendars or family planners I write down this appointment in there too. I know that this may not work for everyone's schedule but on days that are extremely busy, I try to either wake up a little earlier or go to sleep later (even 15 or 30 minutes before/after my usual time) to allow for my self-care ritual. There are sometimes that

I may not be able to do everything in my self-care routine and that's okay we are not perfect but what matters is that we are being consistent and trying our best. If you already have a self-care routine but feel like it is not serving you the way it used to, try to evaluate or see if there are some other things you can remove or include something new to try. The beauty of a self-care ritual is that it is not entirely set in stone. It can always fluctuate and be flexible with any changes throughout your life but as long as it's something that brings you joy and you look forward to then that is all that matters.

14

Conclusion

There you have it! Those are all of the eight types of self-care and some of the best practices that I feel are fitting for each one. Again, there are many more of them out there so please don't feel that you only have to do the ones I discussed. I hope you have enjoyed reading all that I have to offer about self-care for women as I have enjoyed writing it! I wish you the best of luck in creating your own self-care ritual! Go for it as you have nothing to lose but so much to gain!

Also if you did find this book to be helpful, I would greatly appreciate it if you left a favorable review for this book on Amazon!